MY CHILD'S
HEALTH RECORD
From Infancy to Adulthood

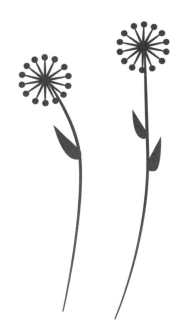

PETER PAUPER PRESS, INC.
White Plains, New York

PETER PAUPER PRESS
Fine Books and Gifts Since 1928

Our Company

In 1928, at the age of twenty-two, Peter Beilenson began printing books on a small press in the basement of his parents' home in Larchmont, New York. Peter—and later, his wife, Edna—sought to create fine books that sold at "prices even a pauper could afford."

Today, still family owned and operated, Peter Pauper Press continues to honor our founders' legacy—and our customers' expectations—of beauty, quality, and value.

Written by Barbara Paulding

Designed by Margaret Rubiano

Copyright © 2016
Peter Pauper Press, Inc.
202 Mamaroneck Avenue
White Plains, NY 10601
All rights reserved
ISBN 978-1-4413-1384-3
Printed in China
13 12 11 10 9

Visit us at peterpauper.com

CONTENTS

Introduction 4

Family Health History................... 5

Notes from Baby's Birth 6

Well Child Visits 8

Sick Child Calls & Visits.................. 37

Record of Illnesses, Allergies, Accidents,
   & Chronic Conditions.................. 48

Immunization Record................. 50

Child's Growth Charts 53

Dental Records.................... 58

Introduction

From your infant's well visits through the first 18 years, record your child's personal health history, with prompted note-taking for well child visits, sick visits, and dental visits, and charts in the back to track immunizations, measurements and percentiles, illnesses, and teething. Record instructions from the doctor (and questions to remember to ask) and more in this handy health journal. With tips and reminders, this little tracker provides the perfect place to compile a clear and concise medical history necessary for school, camp, college, insurance, a change of doctors, and personal reference.

Child's Full Name

Pediatrician's Name & Contact Information

Family Health History

MOTHER'S FAMILY: GENETIC OR MEDICAL CONDITIONS

Name   Relation   Condition & date of onset

FATHER'S FAMILY: GENETIC OR MEDICAL CONDITIONS

Name   Relation   Condition & date of onset

Notes From Baby's Birth

Due date

Date of birth

Time of birth

Place of birth

Doctor

Weight   Length

Circumference of head

Circumference of chest

APGAR at 1 minute

APGAR at 5 minutes

Blood type

Birthmarks

Hair description

Complications of pregnancy

Other notes about birth

Discharge notes

Who to call with questions

Restrictions on food or medicine

Special instructions

Other questions and concerns

Well Child Visits

Pediatricians' schedules may vary and recommendations may change, but generally regular doctor visits are recommended for the following intervals beginning from a few days from birth:

• 2 to 5 days	• 6 years
• 1 month	• 7 years
• 2 months	• 8 years
• 4 months	• 9 years
• 6 months	• 10 years
• 9 months	• 11 years
• 1 year	• 12 years
• 15 months	• 13 years
• 18 months	• 14 years
• 2 years	• 15 years
• 2-½ years	• 16 years
• 3 years	• 17 years
• 4 years	• 18 years
• 5 years	

Of course, any time your child seems ill or whenever you are worried about your baby's health or development, call or visit a health care provider.

Also, use the write-in Immunization Record on pages 50-52, and the Growth Charts on pages 53-57, to keep a shorthand history of vaccinations and growth.

Well Child Visit

Date and time

Doctor

Age

Weight   Percentile

Length   Percentile

Head circumference   Percentile

Immunizations

Tests ordered/results

Questions, concerns, and instructions

Next appointment

Well Child Visit

ONE MONTH OLD

Date and time

Doctor

Age

Weight   Percentile

Length   Percentile

Head circumference   Percentile

Immunizations

Tests ordered/results

Questions, concerns, and instructions

Next appointment

Well Child Visit

TWO MONTHS OLD

Date and time

Doctor

Age

Weight   Percentile

Length   Percentile

Head circumference   Percentile

Immunizations

Tests ordered/results

Questions, concerns, and instructions

Next appointment

Well Child Visit

FOUR MONTHS OLD

Date and time

Doctor

Age

Weight   Percentile

Length   Percentile

Head circumference   Percentile

Immunizations

Tests ordered/results

Questions, concerns, and instructions

Next appointment

Well Child Visit

Date and time

Doctor

Age

Weight   Percentile

Length   Percentile

Head circumference   Percentile

Immunizations

Tests ordered/results

Questions, concerns, and instructions

Next appointment

Well Child Visit

Date and time

Doctor

Age

Weight   Percentile

Length   Percentile

Head circumference   Percentile

Immunizations

Tests ordered/results

Questions, concerns, and instructions

Next appointment

Well Child Visit

Date and time

Doctor

Age

Weight   Percentile

Length   Percentile

Head circumference   Percentile

Immunizations

Tests ordered/results

Questions, concerns, and instructions

Next appointment

Well Child Visit

Date and time

Doctor

Age

Weight .... Percentile

Length .... Percentile

Head circumference .... Percentile

Immunizations

Tests ordered/results

Questions, concerns, and instructions

Next appointment

Well Child Visit

Date and time

Doctor

Age

Weight   Percentile

Length   Percentile

Head circumference   Percentile

Immunizations

Tests ordered/results

Questions, concerns, and instructions

Next appointment

Well Child Visit

TWO YEARS OLD

Date and time

Doctor

Age

Weight   Percentile

Height   Percentile

Immunizations

Tests ordered/results

Questions, concerns, and instructions

Next appointment

Well Child Visit

Date and time

Doctor

Age

Weight   Percentile

Height   Percentile

Immunizations

Tests ordered/results

Questions, concerns, and instructions

Next appointment

Well Child Visit

THREE YEARS OLD

Date and time

Doctor

Age

Weight   Percentile

Height   Percentile

Immunizations

Tests ordered/results

Questions, concerns, and instructions

Next appointment

Well Child Visit

Date and time

Doctor

Age

Weight   Percentile

Height   Percentile

Immunizations

Tests ordered/results

Questions, concerns, and instructions

Next appointment

Well Child Visit

Date and time

Doctor

Age

Weight   Percentile

Height   Percentile

Immunizations

Tests ordered/results

Questions, concerns, and instructions

Next appointment

Well Child Visit

SIX YEARS OLD

Date and time

Doctor

Age

Weight   Percentile

Height   Percentile

Immunizations

Tests ordered/results

Questions, concerns, and instructions

Next appointment

Well Child Visit

Date and time

Doctor

Age

Weight   Percentile

Height   Percentile

Immunizations

Tests ordered/results

Questions, concerns, and instructions

Next appointment

Well Child Visit

EIGHT YEARS OLD

Date and time

Doctor

Age

Weight   Percentile

Height   Percentile

Immunizations

Tests ordered/results

Questions, concerns, and instructions

Next appointment

Well Child Visit

NINE YEARS OLD

Date and time

Doctor

Age

Weight   Percentile

Height   Percentile

Immunizations

Tests ordered/results

Questions, concerns, and instructions

Next appointment

Well Child Visit

Date and time

Doctor

Age

Weight   Percentile

Height   Percentile

Immunizations

Tests ordered/results

Questions, concerns, and instructions

Next appointment

Well Child Visit

ELEVEN YEARS OLD

Date and time

Doctor

Age

Weight   Percentile

Height   Percentile

Immunizations

Tests ordered/results

Questions, concerns, and instructions

Next appointment

Well Child Visit

TWELVE YEARS OLD

Date and time

Doctor

Age

Weight   Percentile

Height   Percentile

Immunizations

Tests ordered/results

Questions, concerns, and instructions

Next appointment

Well Child Visit

THIRTEEN YEARS OLD

Date and time

Doctor

Age

Weight   Percentile

Height   Percentile

Immunizations

Tests ordered/results

Questions, concerns, and instructions

Next appointment

Well Child Visit

Date and time

Doctor

Age

Weight   Percentile

Height   Percentile

Immunizations

Tests ordered/results

Questions, concerns, and instructions

Next appointment

Well Child Visit

Date and time

Doctor

Age

Weight   Percentile

Height   Percentile

Immunizations

Tests ordered/results

Questions, concerns, and instructions

Next appointment

Well Child Visit

Date and time

Doctor

Age

Weight   Percentile

Height   Percentile

Immunizations

Tests ordered/results

Questions, concerns, and instructions

Next appointment

Well Child Visit

Date and time

Doctor

Age

Weight   Percentile

Height   Percentile

Immunizations

Tests ordered/results

Questions, concerns, and instructions

Next appointment

Well Child Visit

Date and time

Doctor

Age

Weight   Percentile

Height   Percentile

Immunizations

Tests ordered/results

Questions, concerns, and instructions

Next appointment

Notes

Sick Child Calls and Visits

You are the first and foremost member of your child's health team. When your child is sick or injured, a call to the doctor's office can help you decide if he or she should be seen by the doctor, or if your child can safely be treated at home. In either case, your records of sick calls and visits—detailing symptoms, diagnoses, treatment, and follow-up—comprise an invaluable medical reference for your child.

Also, use the write-in chart on pages 48-49 to keep a shorthand history of illnesses, allergies, accidents, and chronic conditions.

Date .... Doctor ....

Symptoms ....

....

....

Diagnosis and treatment ....

....

....

....

Follow-up ....

....

Date   Doctor

Symptoms

Diagnosis and treatment

Follow-up

Date   Doctor

Symptoms

Diagnosis and treatment

Follow-up

Date

Doctor

Symptoms

Diagnosis and treatment

Follow-up

Date

Doctor

Symptoms

Diagnosis and treatment

Follow-up

Date   Doctor

Symptoms

Diagnosis and treatment

Follow-up

Date   Doctor

Symptoms

Diagnosis and treatment

Follow-up

Date .... Doctor ....

Symptoms ....

....

....

Diagnosis and treatment ....

....

....

Follow-up ....

....

Date .... Doctor ....

Symptoms ....

....

....

Diagnosis and treatment ....

....

....

Follow-up ....

....

Date   Doctor

Symptoms

Diagnosis and treatment

Follow-up

Date   Doctor

Symptoms

Diagnosis and treatment

Follow-up

Date

Doctor

Symptoms

Diagnosis and treatment

Follow-up

Date

Doctor

Symptoms

Diagnosis and treatment

Follow-up

Date   Doctor

Symptoms

Diagnosis and treatment

Follow-up

Date   Doctor

Symptoms

Diagnosis and treatment

Follow-up

Date   Doctor

Symptoms

Diagnosis and treatment

Follow-up

Date   Doctor

Symptoms

Diagnosis and treatment

Follow-up

Date   Doctor

Symptoms

Diagnosis and treatment

Follow-up

Date   Doctor

Symptoms

Diagnosis and treatment

Follow-up

Date .... Doctor ....

Symptoms ....

....

....

Diagnosis and treatment ....

....

....

....

Follow-up ....

....

Date .... Doctor ....

Symptoms ....

....

....

Diagnosis and treatment ....

....

....

....

Follow-up ....

....

Record of Illnesses, Allergies, Accidents, & Chronic Conditions

DATE   AGE   DESCRIPTION

Immunization Record

VACCINE	DATE GIVEN	NOTES

Hepatitis B

HepB (1)

HepB (2)

HepB (3)

Rotavirus

RV (1)

RV (2)

RV (3)

Diphtheria, tetanus, pertussis

DTaP (1)

DTaP (2)

DTaP (3)

DTaP (4)

DTaP (5)

Tetanus, diphtheria, pertussis

Tdap

***Haemophilus influenzae* type b**

Hib (1)

Hib (2)

Hib (3)

Hib (4)

Polio

IPV (1)

IPV (2)

IPV (3)

IPV (4)

Pneumococcal

PCV (1)

PCV (2)

PCV (3)

PCV (4)

Measles, mumps, rubella

MMR (1)

MMR (2)

Varicella

Varicella (1)

Varicella (2)

Hepatitis A

HepA (1)

HepA (2)

Influenza (yearly)

Influenza

Influenza

Influenza

Influenza

Influenza

Influenza

Influenza

Influenza

Influenza

Influenza

Influenza

Influenza

Influenza

Influenza

Influenza

Influenza

Influenza

Influenza

Meningococcal conjugate

MCV4

Booster

Human papillomavirus

HPV (1)

HPV (2)

HPV (3)

Other

Other

Other

Child's Growth Charts

Although "normal" weight and height of children vary naturally, it's important to monitor your child's growth. The goal is to ensure that the child is consistently within the wide range of normal (between the 10th and 90th percentiles), and that he or she stays on (or close to) the same percentile line over time.

Using weight and length/height measurements from your child's well visits to the doctor, in the charts that follow, find the child's age (across the top and bottom), and length/height and weight (along each side), and mark dots where the age and measurements converge. The curving lines indicate your child's percentile relative to the general population of children the same age.

These growth charts—two for boys and two for girls—from the Centers for Disease Control and Prevention incorporate the latest data from the World Health Organization.

BOYS, BIRTH TO 2 YEARS (LENGTH AND WEIGHT)

Birth to 24 months: Boys
Length-for-age and Weight-for-age percentiles

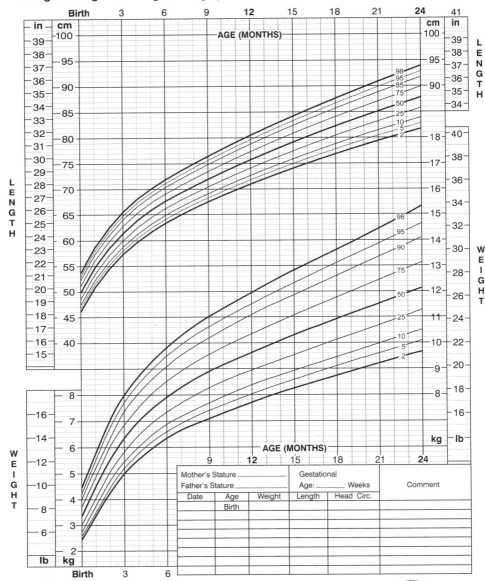

BOYS, 2 TO 20 YEARS (HEIGHT [STATURE] AND WEIGHT)

2 to 20 years: Boys
Stature-for-age and Weight-for-age percentiles

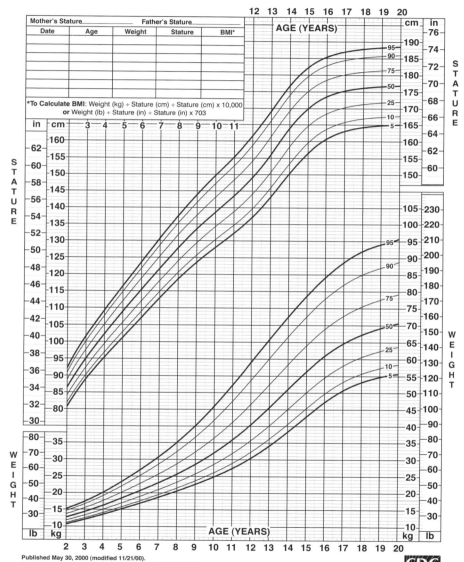

Published May 30, 2000 (modified 11/21/00).
SOURCE: Developed by the National Center for Health Statistics in collaboration with
the National Center for Chronic Disease Prevention and Health Promotion (2000).
http://www.cdc.gov/growthcharts

CDC
SAFER·HEALTHIER·PEOPLE™

GIRLS, BIRTH TO 2 YEARS (LENGTH AND WEIGHT)

Length-for-age and Weight-for-age percentiles

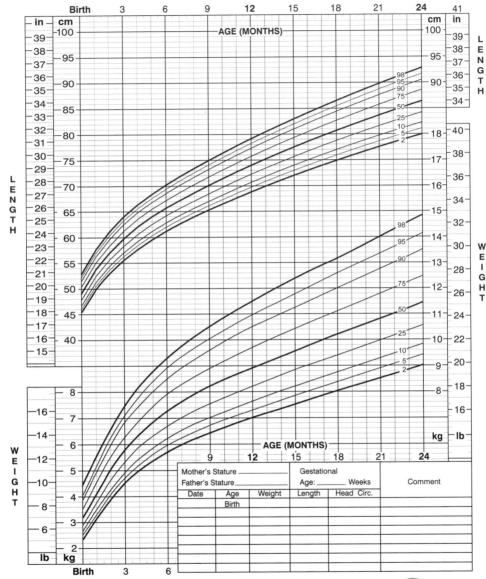

Published by the Centers for Disease Control and Prevention, November 1, 2009
SOURCE: WHO Child Growth Standards (http://www.who.int/childgrowth/en)

GIRLS, 2 TO 20 YEARS (HEIGHT [STATURE] AND WEIGHT)

2 to 20 years: Girls
Stature-for-age and Weight-for-age percentiles

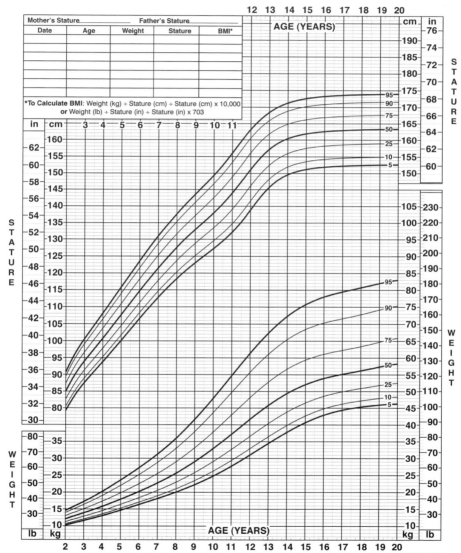

Published May 30, 2000 (modified 11/21/00).
SOURCE: Developed by the National Center for Health Statistics in collaboration with
the National Center for Chronic Disease Prevention and Health Promotion (2000).
http://www.cdc.gov/growthcharts

SAFER·HEALTHIER·PEOPLE™

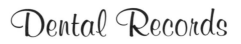

DENTAL VISITS

Dental checkups should take place every 3 months to once a year, as recommended by the dentist. You may consider bringing the child to a pediatric dentist who specializes in children.

DATE	REASON FOR VISIT	RESULTS OF VISIT

Dental care is an essential part of a good overall health plan. It's recommended that your child's first visit to the dentist take place by the time they turn one. The dentist will examine the child's mouth and explain proper oral hygiene practices, including regular brushing, limiting sugary foods, and regular visits to the dentist.

QUESTIONS, CONCERNS, INSTRUCTIONS

DATE	REASON FOR VISIT	RESULTS OF VISIT

Primary Teeth Chart

ERUPTION (MONTH)

SHEDDING (YEAR)

DATE LOST:

DATE APPEARED:

LEFT · RIGHT · RIGHT · LEFT

Upper

Lower

Central incisor (6-7)
Lateral incisor (7-8)
Canine/cuspid (10-12)
First molar (9-11)
Second molar (10-12)

Second molar (10-12)
First molar (9-11)
Canine/cuspid (9-12)
Lateral incisor (7-8)
Central incisor (6-7)

Central incisor (8-12)
Lateral incisor (9-13)
Canine/cuspid (16-22)
First molar (13-19)
Second molar (25-33)

Second molar (23-31)
First molar (14-18)
Canine/cuspid (17-23)
Lateral incisor (10-16)
Central incisor (6-10)

Notes

Notes